Conquering the Course

Obstacle Racing Fitness and Nutrition

Table of Contents

Chapter 1. Introduction

Ready to conquer your next obstacle course race? In our Special Report, "Conquering the Course: Obstacle Racing Fitness and Nutrition," we dive deep into the heart of the thrilling world of obstacle racing. This comprehensive guide isn't just about running, climbing, and jumping - it's a complete overview on physical preparation and nutritional strategies you need to storm through any obstacle course. Whether you're taking on your first race or looking to shave time off your personal best, this report is made for you. We promise an exhilarating read filled with tools, tips, and techniques that will power you across the finish line like never before. So tie your laces and gear up, the race to your next personal achievement begins here! Come, let's conquer the course together!

Chapter 2. Setting the Pace: An Introduction to Obstacle Racing

Obstacle racing is not a simple aerobic dance in your gym, nor is it your neighborhood routine morning run. It's an intense, all-encompassing physical task that pushes your limits in strength, resistance, speed, agility, and quick-thinking. It's not just a race against time, but also a contest with yourself - a ceremonial commitment to breaking barriers, overcoming obstacles, and exploring the boundaries of human potential.

2.1. What is Obstacle Racing?

An obstacle race is a sporting event in which participants overcome various physical challenges. These include running, climbing, jumping, crawling, and balancing elements with the aim of testing speed and endurance. Sometimes referred to as 'adventure racing' or 'mud running,' these races have both natural and man-made obstacles, forcing the competitors to adapt quickly and continue despite the physical demands and harsh conditions.

The origins of obstacle racing are arguably rooted in military training exercises, where soldiers were tested for physical endurance and mental resilience by navigating through challenging terrains with multiple hurdles. In recent years, this grueling sport has leapt from the barracks onto the world stage, with races like the Tough Mudder, Spartan Race, and the Warrior Dash garnering millions of participants and spectators worldwide.

What sets obstacle racing apart from other physical activities or sports events is its unique combination of physical and emotional elements. The thrill of overcoming an obstacle, the camaraderie among racers, the raw grit, and the endearing sense of accomplishment are experiences that make this audacious sport immensely popular and addicting.

Running is the backbone of this sport - it's the stitch that threads the challenges together. Yet, the need to overcome hurdles presents an element of surprise, making endurance and strength training essential for potential racers.

2.2. Training Essentials: Speed, Strength, Endurance, Agility

Success in obstacle racing hinges on training. Since the nature of the sport involves running intertwined with physical challenges, you need to prepare yourself with a multifaceted training regime.

Your performance in obstacle racing heavily relies on your cardiovascular fitness. This is because running is a fundamental aspect of the race, and having a strong cardiovascular base is critical. Long runs, interval training, and hill repeaters are various methods to build cardiovascular endurance. Also, training your leg muscles for long runs will make a world of difference on the race day.

Moreover, strength training becomes vital because of the various physical hurdles you face. This includes climbing over walls, carrying heavy loads, and scrambling under barbed wires. Implementing calisthenics, weight training, grip strength exercises, and body-weight exercises can increase your overall body strength and help you conquer these obstacles effortlessly.

Flexibility and mobility also play a key role in obstacle racing. You need to have the ability to move your body freely, especially when you encounter hurdles that require crawling or climbing.

2.3. Choosing the Race: From Fun Runs to Ultra Marathons

Choosing the right race for you may seem daunting - especially with a myriad of options available. From a 5K 'fun run' festooned with insta-worthy obstacles to the hardcore 24-hour endurance tests, the obstacle races present a full spectrum of challenges.

If you're a beginner, it's advisable to start with a shorter distance race, such as a 'fun run' or a 5K obstacle race. This gives you a taste of what to expect, allows you to assess your skill and strength, and most importantly, helps you understand your areas of improvement. The most important part of these races is to have fun and enjoy the experience!

As you gain confidence and experience, you can take on longer and more demanding races such as the 10K, half marathon, or even ultra marathon races. These races not only test your physical capacity but also challenge your mental toughness, resilience, and determination.

2.4. The Challenge Ahead

Now that you have an introduction to the world of obstacle racing, remember, this is not just about fitness - it's a lifestyle. It represents a commitment to breaking barriers, pushing limits, and challenging the status quo. As any experienced racer will tell you, once you dive in, there's no looking back. You may succeed or stumble, storm through or stagger, but that's the beauty of this audacious sport. It's about learning and growing with each struggle.

The journey that lies ahead will be enduring but exhilarating. It will call upon every ounce of your tenacity and strength. It will break, and then build, your spirit and resilience. So take the leap, brace up, and set the pace. The conquest of your next obstacle race begins now.

Chapter 3. Building Your Physical Arsenal: Strengthening and Endurance Training Guide

Training for an obstacle course race is not only about improving your general fitness level but also sharpening specific skills that match the nature of the course. It's about building a robust and multi-faceted physical arsenal that includes power, endurance, flexibility, speed, agility, and balance. Given that each of these areas is crucial for your performance, we'll cover comprehensive training strategies for each to ensure your success in conquering the course.

3.1. Physical Fitness Basics for Obstacle Course Racing

Firstly, obstacle course racing requires a well-rounded fitness foundation. Hence, regular full-body workouts should be the cornerstone of your training. Here, we'll guide you through the basics of a balanced physical training regimen.

1. Cardiovascular endurance: Make cardio exercises like running, cycling, swimming, or rowing part of your routine. These exercises should vary in intensity and duration, with a typical mix of high-intensity interval training (HIIT), steady-state cardio, and some variation of tempo or threshold workouts.

2. Muscular strength: Incorporate "compound movements," which are those that utilize multiple muscles at once. Exercises such as lunges, squats, deadlifts, push-ups, and pull-ups are excellent choices to build body strength.

3. Mobility: Never overlook the importance of mobility and flexibility. Regular stretching exercises and yoga can greatly improve your overall mobility.

4. Functional training: Mimic common obstacle course movements in your workout for functional fitness. Think burpees, mountain climbers, box jumps, and rope climbing.

3.2. Endurance Training: Building the Stamina to Overcome

Next, let's focus on endurance building, which is vital for maintaining your energy throughout the obstacle course race. Here's a breakdown of routines for each week.

Week 1 – 3: Aim for three days of cardio per week. This could be running or swimming, choosing distances that challenge you but that you can maintain for a longer duration. Always remember to warm-up before running and cool down post-workout.

Week 4 – 7: Now, add interval training to your routine. This might include hill sprints or sprint interval training (SIT), where you'd typically rotate between high-intensity bursts of speed and fixed periods of low-intensity exercise or rest.

Week 8–11: For the next phase, try high-intensity interval training. This could include workouts like running at top speed for one minute, then jogging for two minutes, and repeating that cycle ten times.

Week 12 – 13: Finally, tapering is key before a race. Reduce the volume of your high-intensity work, while maintaining the frequency of your workouts. Focus on resting and rejuvenation.

3.3. Strengthening Workout: Adding Power to Your Arsenal

Strength training is an inevitable part of your physical preparation for obstacle course racing. Here's a progressive strengthening workout plan to add power and strength.

Week 1 – 3: Start with bodyweight exercises that work your entire body, such as push-ups, pull-ups, squats, lunges, and planks. Work on these exercises three days per week.

Week 4 – 7: Incorporate weights into your routine. Begin with lighter weights and higher repetitions, gradually increasing the weights as your strength improves.

Week 8 – 11: Now, focus on challenging compound movements like deadlifts, presses, and kettlebell swings. Maintain three days a week of weight training, while including enough rest for muscle recovery.

Week 12 – 13: Same as with endurance training, opt for tapering towards the end. Maintain the frequency of your workouts but decrease the volume.

3.4. Combining Strength and Endurance Training

As the race day draws closer, it is crucial you learn to handle the physical demands of the course by combining strength and endurance work in the same session. Incorporate routine methods such as the alternating sets method, the circuit training method, or the high-intensity interval resistance training method into your workout.

Don't forget: a successful obstacle course race training program must consider the need to balance stress and recovery. Getting enough rest, hydration, and proper nutrition is just as important as your workout routine. With all these pieces together, building your physical arsenal is within your arm's reach!

Remember, everyone starts somewhere and every step you take brings you closer to your goal. Be diligent, be patient, and be flexible. Get ready to conquer that course like never before!

Chapter 4. Scaling the Walls: Techniques for Obstacle Mastery

Obstacle course races make a point of testing your all-around fitness. In no part of the course is this more noticeable than when you come face-to-face with a towering wall. Without the right technique and strength, these obstacles can be race stoppers. But with the right skills and strategies, they become just another step towards your finish line glory. In this section, we're going to dive deep, breaking down the best techniques to scale walls.

4.1. Building the Foundation: Physical Preparation and Strength

The first step to successful wall scaling is preparation. Wall obstacles put massive demands on muscles all over your body, including your core, upper body, and lower body. Your training program should include a blend of strength training, flexibility exercises, and cardiovascular conditioning.

Bulk up on burpees, pull-ups, and push-ups to build upper body strength as they work out the muscles you'll need to pull yourself up. Develop your lower body and simplify the jumping part with squats and lunges. The plank is effective for the core strength required to lift your legs over the wall. Flexibility exercises help in reducing injury risks and enhance your body's functionality in overcoming walls.

4.2. Hitting the Ground Running: Approach and Launch Technique

How you approach the wall decides how successfully you conquer it. Running at full speed will provide power but smash into the wall and you risk injury. You should approach the wall at a steady jog, keeping your eye on the exact point you aim to grab.

The last few steps before the wall are crucial. You need to transition from horizontal velocity to vertical lift. Putting a bit of an extra push in that last step, you go into a speed squat and then explode upwards, swinging one foot up on the wall for a bit of an extra upward push. If the wall is short enough, this might be all you need.

4.3. Going Up: Climbing over the Wall

Not all walls are small, and even if they were, it's still wise to know how to get yourself up if you miss the grab or slip off. Extend your arms completely; one hand may be slightly higher than the other. This will give you a strong, stable position to bring your legs up.

The most efficient way to bring your legs up is by using the 'heel hook' technique. Raise one leg and hook it over the edge of the wall using the heel of your foot. This shift of weight allows you to pull yourself up with a little less arm strength, thus conserving energy. From this position, you can swing your other leg over the wall.

4.4. Coming Down: Safely Descending off the Wall

Getting to the top is only half the challenge. Now you have to get back down safely. The easiest way is to simply swing both legs over the side and hang, lowering yourself slowly. If you are in a race, however, where seconds count, you may opt to kick off the wall as you swing your legs over, soaring into the air and preparing for a 'parkour roll.'

4.5. Variations and Advanced Techniques

Once the basic wall-climbing techniques have been mastered, you can begin to experiment with variations. Arm strength can be conserved by using 'the mantling' technique. It involves getting your forearm on top of the wall rather than your hand, and then using it like a lever to get your body up and over.

Another advanced technique is 'the cat grab.' This is where you approach the wall at a run, plant both feet squarely on the wall, and allow momentum to carry you upwards as you grab the top with your hands. The benefit of this technique is that it's quick, but it does require precision and an excellent sense of timing.

With a mix of strength, agility, and mental resilience, you can conquer the seemingly indomitable walls on your obstacle course race. These techniques are meant to guide you and acts as building blocks. But remember, every course is unique; every wall different. Experiment with these techniques, adapt according to your body and demands of the course, and make the race truly your own.

Chapter 5. On Your Mark: Pre-Race Preparation and Strategies

The beginning of any hurdle-filled adventure is as important as the journey itself. The commencement of your racing journey isn't necessarily the blast of the starting pistol, but rather your decision to take the leap and plunge into the world of obstacle racing. As such, the pre-race stages are critical to your success. This phase involves physical and mental preparation, equipment choice, nutrition intake, and fostering a winning mindset.

5.1. Physical Conditioning

Physical conditioning isn't about gunning for the first place initially, but gradually improving endurance, strength, and agility. The goal is to finish the race and most importantly, to enjoy the battle with the course. Mark off these essential elements in your physical conditioning:

1. **Endurance Training**: This includes long-distance running and high-intensity interval training (HIIT). Intersperse your running sessions with periods of walking to practice for the stops and starts in obstacle racing.

2. **Strength Training**: Focus on exercises that target your core, upper body, and grip. Examples include pull-ups, push-ups, deadlifts, and farmers walks.

3. **Agility Training**: Obstacle racing demands quick reaction times and adaptability. Incorporate agility ladders, box jumps, and plyometric exercises into your regime.

4. **Flexibility**: Maintain a regular stretching regimen to minimize

the risk of injury.

5.2. Mental Preparation

Mental preparation is as crucial as physical training. It's the key to overcoming the unexpected challenges and maintaining steadiness throughout the race.

1. **Visualization**: Imagine yourself navigating through the obstacles successfully. This creates a blueprint of success within your mind.

2. **Mental Toughness**: Exercises that push you past your comfort zone can help cultivate mental resilience.

3. **Rest and Recovery**: Ensure adequate rest days and practice mindfulness to neutralize stress.

5.3. Choosing the Right Gear

The right gear can make a big difference in your racing experience.

1. **Footwear**: Opt for shoes with a good grip, minimal absorption, and a decent fit.

2. **Clothing**: Opt for moisture-wicking and quick-drying clothes.

3. **Protection**: Consider wearing gloves for better grip, as well as shin and arm guards to prevent scrapes and cuts.

5.4. Race Day Nutrition

Fueling your body correctly prior to the race is integral to maintain energy levels throughout.

1. **1-2 Weeks before Race**: Aim to fill your diet with complex carbohydrates for sustained energy and include lean proteins to aid muscle recovery.

2. **Night before Race**: Opt for a carb-rich meal. Steer clear of high-fiber and fatty foods.

3. **Morning of Race**: Have a light, easily digestible meal like a banana or a slice of toast with jelly.

4. **Hydration**: Start hydrating several days before the race. On race day, sip water regularly but avoid overhydrating.

5.5. The Winning Mindset

Quelling your apprehensions about the race is key to tackling the course with confidence.

1. **Set Personal Goals**: Setting attainable goals can provide a sense of direction and motivation.

2. **Stay Positive**: Maintain a positive mental attitude. Celebrate small victories, and treat setbacks as learning experiences.

3. **Embrace the Unknown**: Prepare to face the unknown and unpredictable. That's part of the excitement of obstacle racing!

Your success in the obstacle course race largely hinges upon your pre-race preparations. Follow these precepts and you're primed for a good performance. Remember, overcoming the course mustn't merely be a quest for the finish line, but an enjoyable journey of learning and growth. Best of luck, and let's conquer this course together!

Chapter 6. The Fuel Factor: Understanding Race Nutrition

Understanding the relationship between nutrition and successful race performance is crucial. It's not just about what you eat on race day, but your overall dietary habits play a significant role in your training, recovery, and performance.

6.1. The Importance of Nutrition

Nutrition is often the missing link in the chain of obstacle racing preparation. When you put your body through the rigorous demands of an obstacle course race (OCR), supplying it with the right fuel becomes even more important. The importance of good nutrition shouldn't be relegated to the days leading up to the race, but understood as a lifestyle to maintain optimal health and performance.

6.2. Macro View: Understanding Macros

Macronutrients are the backbone of any nutritious diet. These are the nutrients your body needs in large amounts and include carbohydrates, proteins, and fats.

Carbohydrates are your body's preferred source of energy, making them essential for any obstacle racer. On the other hand, proteins provide the tools for muscle recovery and growth - they build and repair your tissues. Fats, while often vilified, provide essential fatty acids and fat-soluble vitamins, help in hormone production, and act as a valuable energy source for endurance events.

6.3. Micro View: Micronutrients Essentials

While macronutrients provide the raw fuel, it's the micronutrients – vitamins and minerals – that are indispensable for many body functions, including energy production, hemoglobin synthesis, bone health, and immune function.

Key minerals like sodium, potassium, and magnesium help in maintaining hydration and muscle functions, while vitamins like vitamin C, E, and B-complex contribute to energy production and protect the body against oxidative stress.

6.4. Hydration: Not Just About Water

Hydration is more than just drinking water. When you sweat, you lose electrolytes, particularly sodium and potassium, which are essential for muscle function and maintaining fluid balance in your body. So, rehydrating means replenishing both fluids and electrolytes.

6.5. Meal Timing: Fuelling before, during, and after the race

The nutritional strategy for the OCR should be divided into three key periods: Pre-race, during the race, and post-race.

Pre-race meals should be high in carbohydrates for fuelling your muscles, moderate in protein for satiety and muscle maintenance, and low in fats and fibers to avoid gastrointestinal distress. If you're used to caffeinated drinks, a cup of coffee could offer an energy boost.

During the race, depending on the race length, hydration and carbs become key. Drinking water alongside sports drinks or consuming gels/chews can help keep energy levels steady.

Post-race meals should focus on replenishing glycogen stores and aiding muscle repair. This is the time to consume a balanced meal with a good mix of carbs and protein, along with lots of fluids to rehydrate.

6.6. Supplements: To Use or Not to Use

While proper whole food nutrition should form the core of your eating strategy, supplements can play a supporting role. Always speak with a healthcare provider before starting any new supplements.

Protein powders can be a convenient source of post-race recovery. Creatine can support high-intensity work during training, Beta-Alanine could help with buffering muscle acidity during high intensity periods, and branched-chain amino acids (BCAAs) can support muscle recovery.

6.7. Nutrition Pitfalls to Avoid

Avoid making drastic changes to your diet close to the race day. Your pre-race dinner shouldn't be the first time you try a new meal. Similarly, on race day, stick to tried-and-tested energy gels or chews to avoid any stomach issues. On longer races, don't wait until you're feeling hungry or thirsty to eat or drink; fuel and hydrate proactively.

This is a glimpse of the significant role nutrition plays in the race preparation and execution. Incorporating these tips and understanding into your training routine will not only increase your race performance but foster long-term health. Now that you've fuelled your body right, you're all set to conquer your next obstacle course race!

Chapter 7. Quenching the Thirst: Hydration for High-Performance

Hydration is the cornerstone of any high-performance fitness regime. It's vital not only for maintaining basic physiological functions, but also for supporting vigorous and strenuous physical activities like obstacle course racing. Let's deep-dive into the essence of hydration, how it affects your performance, and the strategies you can employ for optimal fluid balance.

7.1. The Critical Role of Hydration

Water is an essential component of our bodies, accounting for about 60% of our total body weight. It plays various roles in maintaining our health and well-being. Water aids in digestion, absorption, circulation, creation of saliva, transportation of nutrients, and maintenance of body temperature. When it comes to high-intensity activities like obstacle course racing, proper hydration becomes even more critical.

During strenuous physical activities, your body temperature elevates. To cool down, it releases sweat, leading to a loss of body fluids and electrolytes. A balance of these elements is vital for muscle contractions, nerve functions, and energy production, all of which are crucial for racing.

7.2. Essential Hydration Strategies

Knowing you need to stay hydrated is one thing, but understanding how to implement it is another. Below are some of the fundamental hydration strategies that can enhance your performance:

1. **Pre-hydration:** Begin hydrating 2-3 days before your race. Aim for at least 8 glasses (64 ounces) of water per day. Including foods high in water content such as fruits and vegetables can also contribute to this total.

2. **Hydration during training:** Hydrate before, during, and after each training session. This helps replace any lost fluids and prepares your body for the next training session.

3. **Race day hydration:** On the day of the race, start hydrating 2-3 hours before the event. Sip small amounts regularly and remember to continue hydration during the race and replenish fluids post-race.

Remember, hydration requirements can differ depending on individual's body weight, the intensity of the activity, weather conditions, and sweat rate.

7.3. Understanding Your Sweat Rate

A key part of your hydration strategy is to comprehend your sweat rate, the amount of sweat a body produces during exercise. Knowing this helps customize your individual hydration plan as it may differ based on the type of activity, duration, weather conditions, your weight, and genetic factors.

To calculate, weigh yourself (ideally without clothes) before and after an hour of hard training, and record the difference in weight. This difference is mainly the fluids lost through sweat. For each pound lost, you need to consume about 16 ounces of fluid.

7.4. Hydration Tools: Drinks, Gels, and Electrolytes

Hydration in the world of sports is more than just water. Various tools are used by athletes to replenish not just fluids but also electrolytes lost during the activity.

1. **Water:** The most basic tool, water, is an excellent choice for short-duration exercises.

2. **Sports Drinks:** For more extended activities, or those more than an hour long; sports drinks can provide a combination of fluids, electrolytes, and carbohydrates.

3. **Energy Gels:** Energy gels tend to provide carbohydrates to fuel extended exercises but lack in electrolytes and fluids. It's best to consume them along with a source of hydration.

Remember to include a balanced intake of electrolytes in your drinks or meals since water alone can't replenish them.

7.5. Recognizing Dehydration

Dehydration can have severe effects on your performance, and by the time you feel thirsty, you are already dehydrated. Common signs include dry mouth, fatigue, headache, infrequent urination, and dark coloured urine.

More severe dehydration can lead to feelings of dizziness, rapid heartbeat, rapid breathing, sunken eyes, and, in severe cases, fainting or unconsciousness. Paying attention to these signs and keeping an eye on your hydration can prevent these conditions and improve your race performance.

7.6. Overhydration: The other side of the coin

Just as crucial it is to guard against dehydration, overhydration can be equally dangerous. Known as hyponatremia, this condition occurs when you drink so much fluid that your body's sodium levels become dangerously low, leading to symptoms ranging from nausea and confusion to seizures and even coma in severe cases.

The trick lies in striking the right balance and ensuring that your body has the necessary fluids and electrolytes it needs to perform without overdoing it. Therefore, understanding your specific needs, sweat rate, and symptoms are essential.

This chapter has broken down the importance of hydration for high-performance athletes, with a focus on obstacle course racing. From understanding the role of hydration, strategies to keep hydrated, to recognizing signs of dehydration or overhydration, being cognizant of your body's needs is the first step in conquering the course. Stay fluid, stay active, and let's conquer the course together!

Chapter 8. Staying Injury-Free: Prevention and Management

In the realm of obstacle racing, collisions, slips, and falls are part and parcel of the experience. Nevertheless, being prepared not only involves physical readiness and nutritional fortification, but also incorporating strategies to stay injury-free. In this segment, we delve into the mechanisms of injury prevention and management that are critical in conquering any obstacle course race.

8.1. Understanding the Risk

An obstacle course race presents various unique challenges, from leaping over walls and climbing ropes to crossing treacherous terrain. Each presents a potential risk of injury, particularly if your body isn't adequately prepared. Understanding these risks is the first critical step in preventing potential injuries.

Body overuse is often a major risk factor, leading to stress fractures, tendonitis, or worse. Additionally, improper training techniques or equipment can expose you to pulled muscles, sprains, or strains. Proper knowledge, preparation, and execution can significantly mitigate these risks.

8.2. Conditioning: An Essential First Step

Physical conditioning is the bedrock of injury prevention. It would be best if you had a robust and extensive training plan that not only builds endurance for running but strengthens your entire body for the rigors of the obstacles.

Strength training is crucial for building muscular resilience and power. Focus on total body workouts that incorporate exercises like squats, lunges, push-ups, pull-ups, or burpees. These exercises not only build strength but also enhance your agility and balance, significantly reducing the risk of falls or slips. Additionally, training with functional movements mimics the demands of an obstacle race, making your body more adapted to the race.

8.3. Importance of Flexibility and Mobility

Besides strength, improving flexibility and mobility is another critical aspect of injury prevention. Tight muscles can limit your movement and lead to muscle strains and sprains. Incorporating stretching and mobility exercises into your routine enhances your flexibility, aids in muscle recovery, and minimizes the risk of injuries.

Dynamic stretching before workouts and races helps to prepare your muscles for the activity. On the other hand, static stretching after the activity can aid in recovery by reducing muscle tension and enhancing flexibility.

Yoga and Pilates are excellent practices to incorporate into your fitness regime for improved flexibility and strength. They target the deep muscles and promote better range of motion, balance, and body awareness, all essential for navigating the obstacle course successfully.

8.4. Right Gear for the Race

Using the right gear is another element of injury prevention. The right pair of shoes can provide ample support, cushioning, and grip, while specialized clothing can protect you against scrapes, bruises, and the elements.

Choose shoes specifically meant for trail running or obstacle racing, as this footwear provides better traction on uneven surfaces, reducing the risk of slipping or twisting your ankle. High-quality anti-blister socks are a good investment as well to save your feet from blisters.

When it comes to clothing, synthetic fabrics designed for athletic use are best, as they prevent chafing and wick sweat away from your body. Gloves can protect your hands from blisters during climbing and gripping obstacles.

8.5. Nutrition and Hydration

Hydration and optimal nutrition are both crucial for preventing injuries. Dehydration can lead to muscle cramps, hampering your performance and increasing the risk of injuries. Regular intake of fluids during your race can prevent these potential issues.

Nutrition plays a pivotal role in muscular healing and recovery. A balanced diet, rich in protein, carbohydrates, and healthy fats, provides the nutrients required for muscle recovery, growth, and strengthening, in turn aiding in injury prevention.

8.6. Injury Management: Essential Tips

Despite all the precautions, injuries can still occur. Knowing how to manage them effectively can make the difference between a minor setback and a full-blown crisis. Understanding the R.I.C.E (Rest, Ice, Compression, Elevation) methodology to manage injuries can make you better prepared.

If an injury occurs, stopping the activity and taking ample rest is the first step. Apply ice to the injured area to reduce swelling and inflammation. Use a compression bandage for additional support and elevate the injured part to help in reducing swelling.

Seeking immediate professional medical help in case of severe injuries is crucial. Timely interventions can significantly affect the severity and duration of an injury, enabling a speedy recovery.

Remember, in any race, your safety comes first. The thrill of finishing an obstacle race should never compromise your health. Respect your body's signals of pain and discomfort, as they may be warnings of an impending injury. Ensuring proper rest, diet, and hydration are a significant part of the narrative of avoiding injury and staying healthy.

The journey to taking on and conquering obstacle races begins with a commitment not just to training hard, but also to training smart. Prioritize injury prevention and management, and you'll be well on your way to crossing that finish line, triumphantly and safely.

Chapter 9. After the Mud: Post-Race Recovery and Recuperation

The moment you cross the finish line of an obstacle course race, drenched in both sweat and glory, you may feel an overwhelming sense of accomplishment. But your journey is not over yet; the real work begins now - the recovery and recuperation process. This phase is critical in minimizing injuries, improving your performance on the next race, and maintaining overall fitness. This chapter delves into the dos and don'ts of post-race recovery, covering various aspects from nutrition to physical therapy, rest, and everything in between.

9.1. Cooling Down Post-Race

Cooling down should ideally begin right from the moment you cross the finish line. Start by pacing around for about 10 minutes instead of standing or sitting down immediately. Gentle movements like walking can assist in gradually reducing the heart rate, allowing your body to adjust superficial blood flow and redistribute it evenly.

Practicing controlled, deep breathing can also help calm your nervous system down. Exhale longer than you inhale; for instance, take a 4-second breath in, hold it for 4 seconds, and then exhale for 6 to 8 seconds. This reduction in heart rate and blood pressure will allow your body to ease into the recovery mode.

9.2. Stretching and Mobility Exercises

After cooling down, proceed to some light stretching and mobility exercises. Stretching aids in reducing muscle tension and increasing your range of motion, while mobility exercises can restore your joint movements that might have been stressed during the race. A comprehensive stretch should cover calves, quads, hamstrings, glutes, back, shoulders, and triceps. Remember, the goal of these initial post-race stretches is not to increase flexibility, but to flush out lactic acid, relieve muscle tightness, enhance circulation, and ultimately start the healing process.

9.3. Hydration and Nutrition

When you finish an obstacle plan race, your body will be in a state of deficit – it needs water, electrolytes, macronutrients, and micronutrients. Hydrate yourself slowly and continuously over the next few hours. Giving your body a steady supply of fluids will help it better absorb necessary nutrients and continue flushing out toxins.

Post-race meals should comprise both carbohydrates and proteins – carbohydrates to replenish muscle glycogen and proteins to assist in muscle recovery. Aim to consume this meal within a 45-minute window from when you finish the race to avail the maximum benefits of nutrition timing. Micronutrients like vitamins and minerals from fruits and vegetables will further expedite the recovery process.

9.4. Rest, Rest and more Rest

Once the initial steps are done, your body needs complete relaxation to recover. Get plenty of sleep in the days following the race. This is when your body works the hardest to repair any damaged tissues and re-establish homeostasis. Make sure to get quality sleep – deep, uninterrupted bouts of sleep that allow your body to cycle through all the different sleep stages. Consider using tools like black-out curtains, ear plugs, or white noise machines to make your sleeping environment as conducive as possible.

9.5. Active Recovery and Cross-Training

While giving your body rest is critical, inactivity should not equate to sitting or lying down all day. Engage in active recovery such as light cardio, walking, or swimming. These less strenuous activities will help keep your blood flowing and promote faster muscle recovery by feeding your muscles with much-needed oxygen and nutrients. Equally beneficial is cross-training, which works different muscle groups, reducing the risk of overuse injuries.

9.6. Physical Therapy and Massage

If you have the resources and time, seek professional help in the form of physical therapists or masseurs. They can help identify and treat muscle imbalances, knots or trigger points that might have emerged after the race. A good massage promotes blood flow, relaxes the muscles, flushes out toxins, reduces aches, and speeds up recovery.

While your experience right after the race might be bittersweet, the sweetness of recovery accompanied by the right measures will reflect in your performance, strength, and endurance in races to come. So, cherish the mud-streaked victory moment and look forward to the next. After all, the race never ends – every finish line is the start to a new race!

Chapter 10. Obstacle Race Gear: Equipment for Ultimate Performance

The right gear can be the deciding factor between crossing the finish line with a triumphant fist pump or trudging back home, wondering what went wrong. This chapter will be a comprehensive guide to selecting the best equipment to guarantee your optimum performance in obstacle races. Every item we recommend is chosen with the end goal in mind - to get you across that finish line faster, stronger, and safer.

10.1. The Distance Decision

An essential first step in choosing your kit is knowing the length of your upcoming race. This consideration will vastly impact your gear selections. Sprint races, typically around 5 km, require less equipment than a full-fledged Beast Race (20+ km). Hence, adjust your gear list accordingly.

10.2. Footwear Finesse

Footwear arguably tops the list of most important gear for obstacle races. After all, you'll be racing on unpredictable terrain that might include mud, rocks, water, and steep hills. Here's what you need to consider while making your shoe selection:

- Grip: You need shoes with aggressive lugs that can sink into the earth, mud, or sand to prevent slipping. Look for a model with grippy rubber outsoles to provide traction even on wet surfaces.

- Drainage: Obstacle courses frequently involve water. Your shoes should have good draining capabilities to prevent water-logging issues that can slow you down and make your race uncomfortable.

- Durability: Your shoes should be robust enough to withstand harsh terrains and impacts. Look for features like reinforced toe caps and durable upper materials that can protect your feet from sharp rocks.

- Fit: Ensure that your shoes fit well to prevent uncomfortable friction and blisters. Make sure there's a slight room at the toes, a snug fit around the heel, and no undue pressure points.

Remember, always break your shoes in with a few light runs before the big race. There's nothing worse than tackling a myriad of obstacles with painful, blistered feet.

10.3. The Right Race Attire

When choosing your race attire, give preference to comfort, utility, and weather suitability.

- Fabric Choice: Opt for materials that are lightweight, breathable, quick-drying, and easy to move in. Synthetic fabrics like polyester and nylon can be a good bet. Avoid cotton as it gets heavy when wet and doesn't dry quickly.

- Top: Consider a compression top. They not only wick away sweat and keep you cool but may also provide minor protection against scrapes from various obstacles.

- Bottom: Same as your top, either opt for compression shorts or running shorts with a liner. Women could opt for leggings or capris for increased skin protection.

- Weather Gear: Gear up according to the predicted weather condition. Always have a light, waterproof jacket on deck when running in colder or wet conditions.

10.4. Gloves: A Handy Addition

Obstacle races involve a lot of gripping, be it climbing ropes, hauling heavy objects, or crawling through mud. A good pair of gloves can protect your hands from splinters, scrapes, and blisters. They can also provide an improved grip on ropes and wet surfaces. Look for light, breathable, quick-drying gloves with reinforced palms and fingertips.

10.5. Essential Extras

Apart from the basic gear, certain extras can have a significant impact on your performance.

- Hydration Pack: Particularly for longer races, staying hydrated is crucial. Look for lightweight hydration packs that do not hinder movement.

- Nutrition: Mid-race fuel like energy gels or bars can be lifesavers, especially for the longer beasts.

- Headgear: A moisture-wicking headband or hat can keep the sun and sweat out of your eyes.

- Gaiters: These are particularly useful in sandy terrains where you want to prevent sand from entering your shoes.

- Knee Pads: These can provide protection while crawling through rocky terrains.

Remember, the best gear is what works best for you. What works for one racer may not work for another, so always test your equipment prior to race day. It's about finding your best fit, which can indeed be a journey. But with the correct gear selection, you can truly conquer any obstacle that comes your way, making every race an unforgettable one. This chapter has hopefully made the process of finding your perfect gear more streamlined and efficient. Harness your potential and unleash your inner beast; remember, the real opponent is the obstacle course itself. Let's conquer it together!

Chapter 11. Staying Motivated: Mental Conditioning and Overcoming Challenges

Staying motivated through the grueling challenge of an obstacle course race is as much a mental game as a physical one. Overcoming the mental hurdles can sometimes be tougher than leaping over the physical ones. So, buckle up as we tread the path of mental conditioning and facing challenges.

11.1. Mental Preparation: Medal or Not, Prepare Like a Winner

One could argue that the race begins long before you cross the start line. Mental preparation is vital for anyone serious about their obstacle course racing (OCR) performance. Understand that OCR isn't about winning or losing. It's about testing your personal limits, finding your grit, and improving every step of the way.

Visualization is a powerful tool used by professionals across sports. It entails picturing yourself successfully overcoming each obstacle with fluidity and strength. Imagine the sensation of your hands as they grip the monkey bars, the sound of your heart pounding as you climb steep inclines, and the sight of the finish line as you majestically leap over the fire pit.

Meditation techniques can be incorporated into your daily routine, even if it's just 5-10 minutes a day. It aids in stress reduction, improving your overall focus, and allowing better mental endurance on challenging tasks.

11.2. Dealing With The Fear of Failure

A fear of failure can be paralyzing, especially when faced with a daunting obstacle or a challenging race. One of the most effective strategies to combat this is reframing your thought processes.

Instead of seeing failure as a negative outcome, view it as an opportunity for learning and improvement. So what if you couldn't scale that wall on your first attempt? Attempting it taught you more about your strengths and weaknesses. Now you know where to channel your training efforts.

Use positive affirmations to program your mind for success. Phrases like "I am capable", "I am strong", or "I am unstoppable" can have a robust effect on your mindset.

11.3. Mental Toughness: Building Resilience

Mental toughness is the skill that enables you to push through when every muscle in your body is begging you to stop. It's about resilience and endurance.

Developing mental toughness calls for consistent effort and focus. It starts with setting clear, measurable, and motivating goals for your performance. Break down your large goal into smaller, achievable targets. Celebrate these little victories to boost your confidence and maintain morale.

Introduce voluntary hardship into your life. Take cold showers, finish that extra rep, wake up earlier than usual. These deliberate discomforts harden you and make you more resilient when it's race day.

Intermittent fasting techniques can translate into mental perseverance during races. Fasting can potentially improve your mental clarity, concentration, and resilience during long races.

Working on your mental toughness extends beyond just your OCR endeavors, presenting you as a stronger individual in all realms of life.

11.4. Staying Motivated: Pushing Past Plateaus

Peaks and valleys are part of any fitness journey. There will be periods when you feel like you're not improving, no matter how much you train. During these times, it's crucial not to let your motivation wane.

Keeping a training log can help you track your progress and note any improvements – no matter how small. Sometimes, change may not reflect in race times but in workout recovery or strength gain.

Seeking the company of like-minded peers can also help. Participating in group workouts, joining an OCR community, or engaging in fitness forums can expose you to new training techniques, keep your regimen interesting, and provide you with a support system.

Remember, plateaus are a natural part of the growth process. The key is to continue putting in the work, even when improvement seems sluggish. In essence, the plateau can sometimes be a mental obstacle that needs overcoming.

11.5. Post-Race Blues: Handling Highs and Lows

It's common to feel an adrenaline high after a race, followed by a sudden crash – popularly known as post-race blues. Recognize this as a normal part of the racing cycle.

Take the time to reflect on your performance and consider your highs and lows. Celebrate your achievements, no matter how small. Also, ponder upon what obstacles you found challenging and plan how to overcome them in the future.

Maintain a healthy, balanced diet and ensure a good sleep schedule to manage mood swings following the race. Most importantly, remember to take time to rest and recover both physically and mentally.

In conclusion, no matter how advanced the obstacle course, the biggest obstacles we face are often in our minds. By training the mind, we can build mental resilience, power through challenges, and stay poised on the path to personal victory.

Remember, the race isn't always won by the swiftest or the strongest, but by the one who keeps running. Your greatest competition is you, your greatest enemy is doubt, and your greatest weapon is a resilient mind. Prepare it, train it, and let it lead you to the finish line.